THE HOLISTIC MOM

A Mother's Journey into Total Wellness for Mother and Children

By

Lavia Graham

ISBN-13: 9798772524251

Library of Congress Control Number: 2021924687

This book is manufactured in the United States of America.

https://www.thewealthofhealth.online/

Editor: Janet Schwind

Cover Design: Jannatul Nisa

Contents

Introduction:

The Journey Begins

Hello, extraordinary mothers. My name is Lavia Graham. Before you dive into this book, I'd like to share a quick background about myself. I'm the creator and owner of The Wealth of Health, a holistic wellness business. My life path and business teach others the importance of caring for the mind, body, and spirit. I'm a positive spiritual influencer, and I shed my light through blogs,

YouTube videos, doula work, and Reiki Energy Healing. I have also led and taught many meditation and empowerment groups. Most importantly, I'm a mother to amazing identical twin boys who light up my world.

I have always had a love for nature, fitness, and peace. It wasn't until I went through a stressful period that challenged my mental health that I found well-being and my calling to share. In my fourth year of college, I went through a period of mental strain, fog, and anxiety. The anxiety manifested from over stimulating my mind through schoolwork and overexerting my body by not resting enough, as well as my unhealthy eating habits. It was an unforgettable experience that I had never experienced before. I was out of alignment, stressed, and living in a state of fear. My thoughts were uncontrollable and persistent, negative and fear-based. Living in a state of fear wasn't like me, and I knew something was going on but I didn't know what. I lacked control over my mind, and it felt like the anxiety was running my emotions and life.

The anxiety went on for about five months, and then it became unbearable. I started having panic attacks in the middle of the night. I woke up feeling like I couldn't breathe with what felt like a heart attack but what were heart palpitations in my chest. It was terrifying that it affected my sleep. Subconsciously I was afraid to go to sleep because I thought I would wake up with heart palpitations again or my thoughts wouldn't shut off. It was countless nights where I would have to call my boyfriend to stay on the phone so I could feel safe to sleep. The lack of sleep only worsened my anxiety and mental health because I wasn't getting restorative sleep. Our body-mind heals through sleep, and if we are not getting enough, then we can't thrive. The panic attack began spilling into my days. I remember driving in my car feeling claustrophobic and scared to be driving. I would have to pull over and regroup to finish the drive. When the anxiety started taking over my days and nights, I knew I had had enough, and I knew something needed to change.

Before I came to that point, I was coping negatively by overeating junk food to battle my uneasiness and nervousness. Then I turned to indulge in drinking and marijuana. For the first time in my life, I heard the voice of the Higher Power while my own will pulled powerfully against it for attention. My higher self was screaming between the compulsive thoughts! She said, Lavia, this is not you, this is not who you are, and there is a way out. I started to listen to my intuition, and she guided me into changing my diet to fresh fruit, vegetables, whole grains, baked chicken, and fish. At that time, I wasn't vegan. My diet transformation was the beginning of my whole life makeover. I noticed the panic attacks ceased when I stopped putting harmful things—both food and substances—in my body. The compulsive thoughts were still there, but I didn't lose hope. My higher self-guided me to natural herbs to heal my brain from overstimulation. I took magnesium,

CBD, and lion's mane! Natural supplements helped me to sleep at night or to calm or slow down my thoughts.

Discovering those natural supplements was a saving grace for me! My higher self said, Sweetie, don't stop here; you are going to be free from anxiety fully. I knew this to be true because I'm not a naturally anxious person. I wasn't satisfied with needing something unnatural to calm my mind or with the continuing negative thoughts. My higher self began speaking into my consciousness again, and she said, Get into reading. Your higher self speaks to you subtly through repetitive ideas. I would keep speaking, "I need to read books" until I finally decided to go to the half-price bookstore. Next, I got the idea of getting a self-help book. I stayed at that bookstore until I found the perfect book. The self-help book helped me to rewire negative thinking, gain peace of mind, and embrace uncertainty. That book brought me into my spiritual awakening, and it was the most blissful feeling in my life. I freed myself from anxiety. I cried tears of joy every day for months. Through gaining power over my thoughts, resting, and changing my diet, the anxiety vanished! This experience taught me the mind, body, and spirits are connected.

The Divine within wasn't done transforming me! When I awakened, synchronicities began to happen. Signs, words, numbers, and people began appearing in my life. That's when I realized God or the Universe wanted my attention. And to this day, I follow all the signs that resonate with higher living in my life. After I freed myself from anxiety, meditation became synchronized for me. I randomly got an email about free meditation classes at my college campus. I went, and it was just the instructor and me. Out of all the people at the college campus, I was the only one to show up. I knew the meditation class was divinely orchestrated just for me to attend. We did a mind-clearing, compassion, and body scan meditation. I cried during the meditation because I hadn't felt that much peace in my life! I knew it was something I needed. Meditation brings the realization of God's nature within yourself. God's nature is peace, love, joy, compassion, openness, bliss, and freedom. I started coming every week until I deepened my practice.

Then the Divine guided me to shed my light and share what I learned. I started a YouTube channel and started talking about holistic living. I shared life lessons on letting go of fear, trusting the Universe, letting go of judgment, and more topics. The more I shed my light; I was healing myself as well. My light brought more self-awareness of what needed to be healed within myself as well. That's when my first ego death happened or when I realized I had an ego. It was challenging to let that false sense of identity go, and I'm still shedding what no longer serves me. Life is a continuously growing and evolving journey. When I realized my darkness, it brought a sense of humility. That we all have scars, flaws, negative habits, and sin. It made me realize that we are all one with light and darkness and all have our journey to walk through this life. The human walk doesn't define any of us because we truly are spirits having human experiences. In this book, we will dive into my personal holistic and motherhood journey.

Chapter 1

It's Time to Be a Mother

My last year of college was a time of endings and new beginnings. I was focused on growing my empowerment classes and finishing my bachelor's in social work. I was also spreading my wings and letting go of my fears. During that period of my life, I began seeing signs of babies everywhere. I'm not sure if I manifested that subconsciously because I had gotten off the birth control pill after four years and was fearful of being pregnant. It also could have been my unborn sons' souls communicating with me, letting me know I was ready for them to enter my world. Maybe both; I was prepared to be a mom. If I weren't, it wouldn't have happened. What's funny is I knew the night they were conceived.

I told my partner I needed a Plan B immediately after sex because we had an issue with the condom during sex. He gave me the money for the next day, but something in my spirit told me not to take the pill. I let him know I chose not to take it. His response was, "We should be good."

I replied with a sarcastic, "Okay." Five weeks later, I missed my period and I knew something was up. I never missed a period since I had started my cycle as a teen. I told my partner, "I think I'm pregnant." At first, he didn't know I was serious. The next day my period still hadn't come. I called him and said, "What if I'm pregnant? I still haven't got my period."

He replied, "Well, that would be too good to be true."

That was a sigh of relief for me because I wanted the father of my children to want to be a dad. That Monday after class, I went to Walmart to buy a pregnancy test. I had no idea which one to buy. I just picked up one that was a reasonable price. I went home and took it immediately. At that time, I was still living at home with my parents.

Of course, as I started to take the test, I hear my mom walk into the house. I had already peed on the stick. Immediately the test was positive! I peed on another test, and again, it was positive. At that moment, my life changed forever. I was pregnant, and I was embarking on my motherhood journey. I went into my room and cried tears of love. I also felt very nervous. I asked myself if I was ready to be a mom, but I knew I was prepared in my heart. I always wanted to be "established" and married before having children. It wasn't the way I planned, but I knew God had a plan for my sons to be in my life. The year before had been the most beautiful, healing, and transformational period of my life. I was in my power and knew I could handle anything. Everything after that period was Divinely guided.

My son's dad came to pick me up later that evening, and I sprung the news on him. It was a beautiful moment indeed. After four and a half years of dating, we couldn't believe we were about to have a baby. At the time, we didn't know we were in for a surprise of two babies. During that time, we were excited but also had so much to plan and do. When you first get pregnant, you immediately think of all that needs to be done and wanting to let your loved ones know. We needed to pick a doctor, tell our family and friends, find a place to stay together, and of course, plan a baby shower later in the pregnancy. My sons' father handled everything very well. We were in a good place in our relationship at the time and knew we were ready for this next chapter in our love. Before telling anyone the big news, I called my doctor to make sure I really was pregnant. Surprisingly when I went, they didn't retest me. The doctor said that if my home test said I was pregnant, then they would send me over to an OB-GYN. My appointment wasn't until I was ten weeks along. It's kind of like I was left hanging by myself pregnant until that first appointment.

I did notice changes occurring in my body immediately after finding out I was expecting. I was extremely sleepy, and I would fall asleep in an instant. My breast and nipples were sore. I didn't have any more sicknesses but did have slight nausea coming and going for a week. The first few weeks I had cravings for fried food before I knew I was pregnant, but that also subsided. I took being pregnant as an honor, and I wanted to make sure I took care of myself and my babies the best way I knew how. I had already had an excellent self-care routine before I got pregnant and continued it throughout my pregnancy. My daily routine consisted of meditation and yoga for twenty minutes every morning. I journaled and thanked the Divine for my life and the honor to be creating life every day. I spoke and wrote positive affirmations over my sons daily. I wrote that my pregnancy would be smooth and easy. I also journaled that my sons were developing perfectly and healthy.

I made sure I was eating nourishing foods. I was a pescatarian at the beginning of my pregnancy. The only form of flesh food I was consuming was fish. I also ate a lot of fruits, veggies, and whole grains. I ate three times a day because I knew I was creating life. I also made sure I didn't take on any stress from anyone. I didn't worry, and I had faith my whole pregnancy. I also rested as much as I could. I would come home between my internship and classes to nap for thirty minutes. I made sure I slept through the night or when I got home. The first trimester takes a lot of your energy. Everyone's pregnancy is different, but around fifteen weeks, I came back to life. That's when the first ends and the second one begins. I heard a lot of moms say they felt better in the second trimester. My self-care routine helped me and my sons thrive my whole pregnancy.

Chapter 2

First OB-GYN Appointment

It was the ten-week mark, and I was excited about my first appointment. It wasn't much; the doctor was just getting me and my partners' demographic and health information. The morning of eleven weeks was my first ultrasound appointment. I was eager to see what had been growing inside me. The appointment began with me and my sons' father going into the ultrasound room. The nurse put the gel on my belly, and I heard a baby's heart; I looked on the screen and said, "Awe, look at my baby!"

"There are two babies!" the nurse replied.

My eyes got big, and I replied, "TWO?" about six times. My sons' dad said "TWO?" multiple times as well! I look again at the screen and, sure enough, two babies were moving and kicking inside my womb. I was so surprised by how fast my babies were developing. That moment was so beautiful, hilarious, and scary at the same time.

Next, I said, "How am I going to take care of two babies?" and I laid back, grabbed my head, and started to cry. The nurse continued talking, but at that moment, everything went in one ear and out the other. I thought I was dreaming. We went back to meet my OB-GYN, and she started talking more, listing all the possible risks of twins. She also asked if I wanted any other screens or tests done on my babies, but I declined. I'd rather have a peaceful pregnancy than stress myself out on the possible things that could be wrong. After we left the doctor, their dad and I were digesting the wonderful and surprising news that we had two babies on the way. We both handled the information as positively as we could. We needed to stick together as soon-to-be new parents.

After processing the news of having twins, we were excited but a little more focused on preparing for our new life. My pregnancy health became even more critical because a twin pregnancy is considered high risk. Not only did I have to keep myself healthy, but I also had to nurture two babies to life. I was up for the double blessings! I didn't let anything the doctors told me make me afraid of carrying my boys full term. My faith and spirituality kicked in. I only spoke, wrote, and claimed what I wanted to happen for my babies. My positive affirmations kept myself and the babies happy, peaceful and growing beautifully. My self-care also became double important! I made sure I kept up my daily routine of healthy diet, body movement, and resting.

Chapter 3

Confidently Sharing Your Pregnancy News

When I found out I was pregnant, I knew I wanted to protect myself and my baby's energy. I wanted to share the news with the individuals I trusted. I also prepared myself for any reaction from others. You get a lot of unsolicited advice and judgments when you become pregnant. Knowing that others are judgmental is why I prepared myself in advance not to be affected by any of their reactions. I made sure I thought positively about my pregnancy experience and considered my pregnancy a blessing. Knowing how others felt wasn't necessary. In the higher scheme of it all, I'm the one living my motherhood journey. I did want to make sure my parents knew because they are the people who matter to me. I was extremely nervous about sharing the news with my parents because I knew they would be surprised. I also knew they wouldn't be happy I got pregnant before marriage. Even though my pregnancy wasn't in the plan, I was not ashamed at all. I didn't want to wait long to tell my parents because I didn't know when my belly would show. Being my first pregnancy, I thought I would show immediately. The funny part is I didn't start showing until almost five months. I told my parents at around six weeks.

I first began by telling my mother. I felt I needed to share the information with her because I knew her reaction would come with some advice. I told her most sporadically. She was walking to the laundry room, and I was sitting in the kitchen and blurted out, "Mom, I'm six weeks pregnant!"

Surprisingly she was calm about it at that moment. I had planned to tell her and my dad at the same time while my partner was there, but I felt I needed to give her a heads up before I did it. It also brought me peace because what women wants to keep that from their mother? After telling my mom, she said that my partner and I need to tell my dad. She arranged the sit-down for all of us to talk and share the news. When announcing your pregnancy news to close loved ones, having everyone there helps. That way, everyone can talk and get everything out at one time. During our talk, my parents wanted to know my partner's plan to provide for the family. They also discussed the seriousness of being parents. I appreciated the discussion but still only took in what resonated with me. After that talk was over, I was relieved. Sharing the news with anyone else didn't bother me as much. When I told friends, I had a nervous feeling, but I was mostly excited. I told two of my friends out at lunch because I like to see others' reactions in person. They were happy for me, but I must warn you: be prepared to answer questions. There will always be tons of questions about your plans, gender, baby's name, etc. Don't feel obligated to share everything; your pregnancy journey is personal.

I didn't share my news on social media for my pregnancy journey's peace and sacredness until my third trimester. Pregnancy is the most life-changing journey. My pregnancy was also considered high risk. For that reason, I wanted to protect my and my unborn sons' energy. Keeping my pregnancy private was the best decision I made. I was able to enjoy and grow my sons beautifully without too much outside energy. I announced my pregnancy two weeks before my baby shower on social media. As I expected, so many commented and said congratulations on the news. A lot of people were shocked I was pregnant with twins. That whole evening my phone was blowing up with comments. At that time, I was emotionally ready to handle it. I would advise all moms to wait until they're emotionally prepared to handle others' comments.

Takeaways:

- Get a list of people who are important to you to share the news with.
- Be prepared for whatever reactions arise from others.
- Be prepared to answer questions.
- Protect your energy by staying peaceful and trusting that you're prepared for your motherhood journey, regardless of others' reactions.

Chapter 4

Mentally Preparing to Be a Mother

Having one baby is hugely life-changing. Having two babies is double that. I knew I had to prepare myself for motherhood mentally. The mental preparation started as soon as I found out I was pregnant. I knew I wanted to handle the journey positively, peacefully, gracefully, and with joy. Gratitude mentally prepared me always to be thankful for the good in my pregnancy and life in general. I knew I wanted to carry that tool into my daily motherhood journey. Gratitude strengthens and trains your subconscious mind to look at the good over the not-so-good. I honestly believe that's why I had such a smooth and wonderful pregnancy. I shifted my mental state immediately when any uncomfortable feeling or thought would arise. Gratitude is also working with the law of attraction to bring you more good. When you're thankful, your aura vibrates higher. Gratitude sends signals out to the Universe to attract more blessings. Meditation was my other daily mental preparation for motherhood; it elevates your whole being and brings peace to your mind. The daily practice of meditation has so many health benefits. It was beautiful meditating during pregnancy because it helped me and my babies bond. It also helped my sons to develop healthily. Meditation helps the body and brain to self-regulate to handle stress positively. It enables the body to rest and repair. Any time I felt tired, I meditated. I constantly meditated for ten to twenty minutes every morning and midday. Meditation helped me to be grounded and full of bliss during my pregnancy. Meditation also increased my energy during pregnancy because it gave my mind and body rest. After my meditation, I would keep the peace and present awareness throughout the day. It mentally prepared my mind to live in the moment. I knew meditation would still be a necessity after my sons were born.

Journaling daily helped me to prepare mentally for motherhood, too. I wrote out daily affirmations that my sons and I were healthy. I also wrote that I would have peaceful and easy children to raise. The journaling was manifesting and creating my reality. My pregnancy was excellent, and my sons are such a joy to raise. Journaling prepared me to expect the good and the best out of motherhood mentally.

I also mentally prepared for motherhood by reading. I acquired as much knowledge as I could through baby apps and reading books. The twin motherhood book helped me prepare for a life with twin boys; it gave me information on the best baby products to purchase for twins. The book also demonstrated breastfeeding techniques and much twin life information. Of course, every motherhood experience is different, but the book gave me a great heads-up on what was important. I truly felt confident and prepared

for my sons.

Chapter 5

Physically Preparing to Be a Mother

Before becoming a mother, I had no idea how much we use our bodies to take care of the babies after pregnancy. Let's not forget the physical strength needed to carry and birth children. A mother needs to be physically healthy and strong throughout her whole motherhood experience. The summer before becoming pregnant, I worked out daily and even did some strength training. I love exercising, but I wasn't intentionally preparing for a twin pregnancy. I subconsciously knew what my body was about to endure, so I prepared. That fall, I decided to become a pescatarian and give up any other meat. I drank more fresh juice and vegetable juices and detoxed my body. Being pescatarian and eating fresh also helped to cleanse my womb of toxins before my pregnancy. I also believe this helped reduce morning sickness because my body already got rid of waste when I changed my diet. I did yoga daily before and during my whole pregnancy. Yoga helps with cultivating peace, lowering stress, strengthening and toning the body. A mother needs to be stress-free to develop a baby or if she is trying to conceive. (Several recent studies have found links between a woman's levels of day-to-day stress and lowered chances of pregnancy. For example, women whose saliva had high alpha-amylase levels, an enzyme that marks stress, took 29 percent longer to get pregnant than those who had less.) https://www.webmd.com/baby/features/inferti lity-stress

Not only is it essential to be healthy to conceive, but it's important to be strong enough to carry the baby or baby's full term. Since I already had a high-risk twin pregnancy, I knew I had to take extra care of myself. In my first trimester, I stuck to light workouts and walking. I didn't have as much energy for challenging exercises because creating my sons took a lot out of me. I also rested a lot. Another way to physically prepare for motherhood is by sleeping. Getting enough rest is essential for the mom to regain her energy during pregnancy and for motherhood. I meditated every morning and afternoon before my nap. I napped daily in the middle of the day on lunch breaks when I was balancing an internship during last semester of college and working during my first trimester. In the middle of my second trimester, I was blessed to stay home while my partner worked. I did work on my business while creating, nesting, and preparing for my sons.

In my second trimester, I had more energy to be more active. Most moms can agree that the second trimester is where you have the most energy. The second trimester is an excellent time to create a workout routine. I did light cardio workouts and ten-pound dumbbells to keep my muscles strong. I only worked out for about 25 minutes and a couple of days a week. I never overdid it. I only worked out enough to get my blood flowing and heart pumping. My morning and evening yogas were usually 15 minutes. It's best not to overexert yourself because it can harm you or the baby.

My diet during pregnancy was pretty healthy. I had a fresh smoothie every morning and some nights, and ate whole-grain waffles with fruit. On days where I was extra hungry, I would eat eggs, toast, and a veggie patty. I ate eggs before I became vegan; they do have plant-based alternatives for eggs now. I would eat baked fish, vegetables, and whole-grain rice for most meals for lunch and dinner. I also loved vegan burritos and chili. Of course, a pregnant mom can eat unhealthy sometimes due to cravings. I had my moments where I craved fried foods or sweets. Don't deprive yourself of a craving, but don't overdo too much processed and junk food. It is essential to be mindful that what you eat nourishes you and develops your baby's mind, body, and energy. I suggest limiting unhealthy snacks or meals to one per day at most. The other meals should be something fresh, healthy, and preferably, home-cooked. The better you eat, the more energy you will have and the happier you will feel while creating life. This energy, happiness, and health will manifest in your

babies.

Chapter 6

Spiritually Preparing to Be a Mother

The year before I got pregnant with my twins was a spiritually enlightened time in my life. I had awakened to my inner light of pure God-consciousness and awareness. Awakening means I remembered that I'm more than just a physical body and my mind. I awakened to my boundless spiritual energy. Your eternal self is God's force within you. Your spiritual energy is the real you, and this God force is within everyone, everything, and beyond. I realized who I genuinely am, and it opened the door to love, joy, peace, bliss, gifts, and everlasting freedom. After I awakened to my light, I experienced an ego death. When you take form into a human form, an ego naturally occurs in the lifespan. The ego isn't all bad, but it can be if you take on its lower vibrational qualities. These qualities are judgmentalness, fear, negativity, and belief in separation. A higher vibrational ego makes choices that will positively elevate self, self-respect, and honoring your truth. When I had ego death, I had to let go of thoughts, fears, and self-judgments holding me back from my light. When I spiritually chose to let go, I felt free internally. I wasn't in bondage to thoughts or insecurities. I ascended spiritually and was shining like never before.

When I connected to my light, my spiritual gifts and intuition grew. The Divine Universe began giving me signs through numbers, synchronicity, and symbols. The divine realm, angels, ascended masters, spiritual guides, and ancestors speak with you through symbols. For example, my angels would use butterflies to get my attention.

Butterflies symbolize freedom and transformation. I could see a shirt with a butterfly on it with a positive message that I needed to see at that moment. A physical butterfly could fly past so that I could touch it. If the butterfly lets me touch it, I know it's a loved one. My spiritual guides would also use owls because that's my spirit animal. When I was going through my spiritual awakening, I would see owls everywhere. I remember looking up what owls symbolized spiritually, and it meant spiritual awakening and transformation. The more you follow your intuition, meditate, live presently, and in a state of peace, you will grow more spiritually.

That period after my awakening, I saw signs about babies. I even questioned if it was time for me to become a mother? It didn't fit in with the "plan" I had for myself. I wanted to be married and well off into my career before becoming a mother. That wasn't God's plan for my life. I saw the baby sign for about five months before I got pregnant. I even knew that night my partner and I conceived our sons. I didn't plan the night, but something told me I was pregnant immediately after having sex with my partner. I wanted to get a Plan B, but my spirit said no. I'm so happy I listened to my heart because God granted me two amazing sons.

Sometimes we take for granted the gift of being pregnant and becoming a mother. If God blesses you with a baby or babies, then it is your time to step up to that purpose.

After getting pregnant, I started seeing signs of boys everywhere. While working at my job at an after-school program, I searched on Google, "How do you know the gender of your baby?" As I typed, I looked up across the room and I saw the word "boy" on the punching bag across the gym. That moment I knew it was a boy, but the Universe saved a surprise of it being two boys until my ultrasound! The day before I found out the gender, I saw two twin boys at the park. On the way to my appointment, I saw a beautiful light, baby blue cloud. It was so beautiful, and I knew the Universe was speaking to me. When I had the gender reveal at my appointment, the nurse asked if I wanted to know the sexes! I said yes, but in my head already knew what my babies were. I looked at the ultrasound and cried. I was really about to be a mother of two identical precious boys!

The miracle of creating life in your body touches your heart far beyond the mind's understanding. From the very beginning of my pregnancy, I spiritually started to prepare myself for this pivotal point in my life. It was no longer just me anymore. I was preparing to nurture three people daily, and four including my partner. It's a time to absorb and connect with the Divine for guidance. Every day I surrender my life over to God fully because having twins wasn't a part of my human vision for myself. I knew there was a deeper meaning for my beloved sons coming into my life at that point. To spiritually prepare for my sons, I meditated daily and was open to insight and signs the Divine gave me. It is so important to sit with God's presence every day. I would spend time in nature to connect with God and feel joy throughout my pregnancy. Spirituality is connecting with the true spirit and happiness within yourself. When I'm outside in nature, I feel spiritually connected to life. The feeling of being connected to nature brings natural joy to my heart.

I also spiritually prepared for my sons through journaling and gratitude. I feel I had a spiritual bond with my sons while they were in my womb, and I always connected with them during times of journaling, prayer, meditation, and gratitude. I always told them I was thankful for them and that they will be such a joy to raise. I knew that all the love I put into them in my womb would manifest into how they are in the world.

Lastly, I spiritually prepared myself for motherhood by planning how I would handle its most challenging days. I already had a mental idea of what I needed to do to stay positive and strong. I told myself I would pray, meditate, and keep positive things on in my background. I would play all my favorite spiritual teachers' sermons on TV in the newborn days of motherhood. It helped me to stay motivated when the fatigue kicked in. I also positively affirmed that I'm strong and counted my blessings all day long. You have to keep your thoughts high to prevent breaking down. Counting your blessings keeps you positive and focused on the present moment. I believe every mom should have some type of game plan on how they will handle stress. The newborn days can get very intense with no sleep in the first few months. I still use the same technique now that my boys are one-year-olds because there are still days in motherhood when you can get tired and need motivation. If you don't take care of yourself for an extended period, it can result in mommy burnout. I feel all mothers go through some mom burnout. That's why it is essential to create a stress relief plan. It will help bring you back in balance—mind, body,

and spirit.

Chapter 7

Preparing Your Home for Baby's Arrival

There's so much to do when preparing for your bundle (or bundles) of joy. Getting your home ready is one of them. First on the list is assessing the security and environment. It is ideal to have your own place to bring your baby home to before getting pregnant—but if that isn't your situation, it's okay. My partner and I were living separately when we conceived, but finding a place to stay, together with our baby, was our main focus as soon as we found out. It is important find a place where you feel comfortable and safe bringing your baby. Also finding a place you can afford is essential; financial planning is a part of security. Having children is expensive, so it is important to make sure you can keep a roof over your head whether you are with your child's father or not. Planning ahead and having a backup plan will create security for your family.

Try your best to get a place to stay before your second or third trimester. Ideally you want to be settled by your second trimester when you have the most energy to unpack and get your place together. It is important to bring your new baby into a clean and uplifting environment. Clear the stagnant energy, making time to get rid of what you don't need in your home. Keep your house as clean as possible because during the third trimester, you're not going to have the energy or desire to do as much.

Start preparing and organizing your baby's room. After the baby shower, the boys had so much to sort and put away. We were blessed to get almost everything we needed from the shower. My living room was filled with baby shower gifts for almost a week. Whenever I had energy I would tackle putting things away little by little. I washed, hung, and sorted their clothes by size. Surprisingly, putting away tiny human clothes is a lot of work! I had their dad move and put together the more challenging gifts.

Sage your home and decorate it with love. I usually keep fresh flowers around and crystals for positive energy. In the third trimester, have your partner or loved one help you deep-clean the house before the baby's arrival. When you come home, all your focus will be able to go straight to the new baby. A clean home is also good to lessen your newborn's exposure to harmful bacteria.

Chapter 8

Bonding With Your Spouse

Bringing new life into the world is a massive change to any relationship. It is so essential to make time for your partner in the midst of preparing for your baby. When I was pregnant, my partner was working a lot, and it seemed like it was a challenge for us to hang outside the house. We did take some time to get out on the weekends, but we were both tired during the week. On our weekends out, we grabbed dinner, went to the park, went to the mall, or went to the movie theater. We also would do simple things together like grocery and baby supply shopping. We had a couple's vacation in mind, but unfortunately that didn't happen.

Bonding with your partner doesn't always mean having to leave the house, though. You can spend meaningful time together at home, as long as you make sure to create a special space to enjoy your quality time. We made time to watch movies together, and I would bake cookies for a special treat. Another way we bonded was with weekly moments of meditation, prayer, and yoga. Holistic practices connected our love spiritually. These moments meant the world to me—and us—because I knew our whole life was about to change.

Once your baby is born, bonding time with your partner becomes even more important—but harder to achieve. There is so much stress surrounding being a new parent and if you are not careful it will subconsciously create a void between the two of you if you don't intentionally make time to connect. Now we live in a pandemic time, which makes it even harder to enjoy date nights. When you go out, you're thinking about your safety. To avoid excessive worry when we go out, I try to live in the moment as much as possible. I also visualize perfect health and safety surrounding us as we enjoy each other. Time alone helps you remember the life you had before the children and the still connection. Date nights are essential when you bump heads, feel pressure, and want to throw in the towel. Nights away or bonding at home helps to restore the union.

It takes a lot of love, prayer, faith, kindness, and communication to keep a relationship alive. Every day, make an effort to say or do something kind for each other. It can be as simple as saying thank you for all you do for this family. Appreciation and communication are essential to each parent as they take on parenthood. Be sure to express what you need and feel. Your partner is not a mind reader, so be open. You can do something kind by giving your partner a hug or a kiss while in passing. Showing affection lowers stress, tension, and distance between one another. Yes, parenthood can be a lot on a couple, but keep your respect and love "on" and you will weather any storm.

Chapter 9

Babies' Arrival

It was my 37th week of pregnancy, and I was just physically "over" the consistent doctor checkups. Since I was carrying twins, I had a regular OB-GYN and a high-risk doctor I saw twice a month during my second trimester and weekly during my last month of pregnancy. The doctors had to watch the babies and me closely to make sure everything went smoothly and well. I was blessed to have a smooth pregnancy, but near the end, mommy was so over it. I was waking up throughout the night to eat and pee. Getting kicked in the ribs and sharing my body with two humans was getting uncomfortable. I knew the boys were ready to come out also. Imagine sharing a womb with a twin brother for almost nine months. It had to be super cramped because I'm a petite lady.

It was Thursday, my last doctor's appointment and ultrasound before my baby's arrival. This appointment was to see if I could have a natural birth. My sons were labeled Twin A and Twin B. Both babies had to be head down, or at least Twin A had to be head down for me to be able to have a natural childbirth. That way, I could push the babies out without complications. I mentally accepted a vaginal or C-section delivery. The high-risk nurse checked my son's positioning, and Twin A was breeched (head up). They were transverse (side-lying) for most of my pregnancy, but Twin A turned breech the last month, and Twin B was transverse. After seeing that A was still breeched, I had peace with having a C-section. I'd rather have me and both my children be safe during delivery than risk one of our lives. I did have an issue that occurred with the guest doctor filling in during my last appointment. Before seeing my babies' ultrasound, I got my blood pressure checked, and it was slightly elevated. Higher blood pressure is common when pregnant with twins, and I monitored my blood pressure to watch for preeclampsia. The guest doctor suggested I needed to have my sons that night, which was overwhelming to me. I wasn't scheduled to have my boys until another week. I asked the doctor if I could wait and talk to my OB-GYN to see her opinion because I'd rather still wait if I could. The conversation then turned into a heated debate. I understood he was a professional, but I felt I wasn't being heard or respected.

The appointment ended with me storming out of the room crying, ready to report the doctor. The doctor was more worried about being correct than comforting an emotional, almost nine-month pregnant mother with twins. Being upset raised my blood pressure even more. If I were to get pregnant again, I would make sure to have outside support always there to advocate for me, or another perspective. External support would be a partner, loved one, or doula. As soon as I walked into the room, I talked to the receptionist about reporting this doctor. The receptionist allowed me to go back and talk to the head of the department. I told the head about my experience. I felt disrespected, unheard, and racially mistreated. The department head told me he (the doctor) was wrong for how he treated me, and handled the situation. After leaving the high-risk doctor, I went to my OB-GYN appointment downstairs on the floor below. By the time I got to my appointment, the high-risk doctor had already contacted my OB-GYN. The OB-GYN agreed with the high-risk doctor that I should have my sons earlier. She even suggested I have my twins that night. Again, I felt overwhelmed and wasn't ready to have my twins that same day. My energy needed to be peaceful and grounded before I could bring my boys into this world. I told her no to that night. Then she suggested two days later, which was a Saturday. My scheduled C-section wasn't until the following Tuesday so I told her I'd think about it. I had my mind set on that Wednesday. She told me she would give me a call on Friday to see how I was doing. I was shocked by my experience with the last doctor and overwhelmed with emotion, but so grateful that the rest of my pregnancy and doctor experience was highly positive.

The next day I took it super easy and rested all day. I could tell my boys were running out of room by them kicking my ribs with such frequency. The boys were also sitting on top of my bladder. And they were taking so much of my energy that all I could do was rest in bed. Spiritually I knew I couldn't stretch the delivery until the following week. Mentally (and due to my pride), I wanted to wait to bring them into the world on the date that I wanted. My doctor called me that evening and told me she already scheduled the C-section for Saturday. I was upset because I still thought I could wait. I called my sons' dad and told him that the doctor wants us to have our twin boys tomorrow. He was surprised and a little anxious also. He left the decision up to me. Before I had called him, I told the doctor I needed some time to think about it because it changed our plans. Instead of me going off emotions, I needed to be logical. Logically and physically, I knew my body was finished with the pregnancy. That morning I also got a spiritual sign. A bracelet I bought at the beginning of my pregnancy was a set of crystals that would protect the mom and unborn babies during pregnancy. It also helped with the babies' development. I wore it every day of my pregnancy. The morning before my doctor called, I woke up to crystal beads broken in my bed. I took that as a symbolic meaning that my sons were ready to come into this physical world.

After I meditated and considered how I felt physically and spiritually, I decided to have my babies the next day. That night was filled with high emotions and some fear. My life was going to change forever. I was going to go through a C-section surgery to meet my sons for the very first time. I was so nervous because I had never been through surgery before where I had to be cut open. Luckily my mother experienced a C-section with two of her three children, so I knew what to expect. My nerves kicked in about getting an epidural. With all the nervousness I began to stop and breathe and affirm that everything would go smooth and amazing. I knew my babies and I would be protected during the delivery process. I also declared that I am stepping into motherhood with ease and grace. My affirmations helped to calm me down. The last night before my baby's arrival was spiritual and sentimental for my partner and me because this was our last night being in the home and together with just him and me. We spent five years of our lives together before having children. He was filled with nervousness and emotions just like I was. It was beautiful; we spent our last night making sure the boys and I had everything we needed in our bags when we arrived home. We went to the store and got snacks and stopped and grabbed food. When we got home, we prayed and went to bed. I couldn't sleep because the boys' movements, excitement, and nervousness were keeping me awake.

That morning we got up at 8 a.m. to get ready to go to the hospital. I started my morning with prayer, meditation, and a shower. My partner and I took many pictures of my last few hours of being pregnant with our sons. It was super sweet! We listened to relaxing R&B music on the way to the hospital. I remember my dad calling me with love and encouragement right before we checked in. I remember saying I will be leaving this hospital with two amazing boys on my way up to the hospital. After getting checked in, my mom, my partner's mom, and auntie were there to comfort us until it was time to deliver our precious boys. A nurse came in and did one last ultrasound to check the positioning of the boys. Unexpectedly we had to wait another hour before we could deliver because my doctor had an emergency C-section to deliver before mine. I was hungry, thirsty, and restless because I couldn't eat or drink until after the delivery due to my C-section.

The hour passed quickly, and it was time for me to meet my sons for the very first time. They walked me back by myself to get my epidural. My partner couldn't come to the delivery room until I got in. Let me tell you that walk to the delivery room was when all my emotions set in. I began to cry; I was walking into my new chapter of motherhood. I felt nervous about getting the epidural, but I knew God and my angels were protecting me. I have an uncle who went missing almost three years ago. Dealing with him being gone was and is very emotional to me because I was close with him. I spiritually know that he has passed on because he gives me signs of his presence daily through numbers, synchronicity, seeing his name, and hearing his name. I remember right before they were about to start the epidural, one of the nurses said, "Nurse Ryan is downstairs." It was no coincidence the nurse said that name. That was my uncle's name. He was spiritually letting me know he wasn't going to let anything happen to me. That moment filled me with so much love and peace.

After the nurse performed the epidural, my partner came in for the C-section. When the epidural kicked in, my body started to go numb. I lay back on the operating bed, and they began the procedure. I began crying when the doctor started cutting me open. Even though I had an epidural, I could still feel the pulling and tugging. My partner was so calm and soothing while the procedure was happening, despite him seeing my whole insides. It didn't take any time for her to pull out my first son Zion. When they pulled him out, he wasn't making noise at first. He was a little bit shocked to come into the world, so they made him make a noise. When I laid eyes on him, I was at a loss for words. I couldn't believe this human being was coming out of my body. One minute after, they pulled out my son Zane; he came out crying. I was in extreme amazement! Two precious boys, two identical twins, just came out of my body so handsome and breathtaking. Both had a head full of hair. The doctor and nurses took the boys over to the scale to weigh them; they both weighed a little over 5 pounds, a healthy size for twins.

My partner went to look over and meet our sons. I wish they would've placed them on me first before they got weighed, but I understood that was an important protocol. But being that I am their mother, I feel I should get the first look at the boys. But it's okay. I spent almost nine months creating them in my body, so we were spiritually connected. When the nurse brought the boys over, the first thing I did was kiss them. I couldn't believe that these extraordinary human beings were created in my body. It was the most powerful thing I've ever experienced in my entire life. My sons were so precious, filled with so much love and peace. The nurse and my partner rolled me to our room so I could nurse the boys for the first time. The hallway was filled with our loved ones greeting us, telling us congratulations on the way to the room.

Some of our loved ones followed us into the room and instantly wanted to hold the babies; we understood they were excited, but I had just met my boys for the first time. I wish I could've had them a little bit longer before I had to pass them over, but the nurses didn't let our visitors stay long because I had to nurse the boys. I didn't have much knowledge of breastfeeding before I started tandem-feeding the boys. I read a bit of it in a book, and I took a nursing class. The class wasn't in-depth, so I just went with the flow of nursing my boys. I used my motherly instincts to get the boys to latch on; to my surprise, both twins latched on immediately. There was a lactation specialist who came in to help me during my first time nursing the boys. She helped me prop the boys up properly during tandem-feeding with pillows.

The first feedings after delivery are colostrum until the breastmilk is entirely in; when I wasn't breastfeeding, I was pumping to gain a milk supply. I had no idea all the work it took to get your breastmilk flowing in. After I finished nursing for the first time, I got to drink and eat again. At first, I was just eating ice chips because that's what I was craving. I was so thirsty, then I ordered room service to get my first meal. The hospital food wasn't that great, but I needed to get something in my body. After I ate I tried to relax and rest for a little bit following my procedure, but I couldn't sleep much because I decided to breastfeed my boys fully. Fully breastfeeding requires you to feed your children every two to three hours. It seemed like that two- to three-hour mark came every thirty minutes!

I tried to nap when I could. My partner and I sent the babies to the nursery when we tried to grab a quick nap. A short rest was what we got. We heard that baby cart roll in and we knew it was time to be in parent mode. My partner was so attentive and helpful with my breastfeeding journey. He would help me prop the babies on my breasts for feeding. When I pumped, he would feed one of the babies with a tiny syringe to help me out! The nurse gave us the idea of using a syringe because babies only drink around 15 ml of milk or colostrum in the beginning. Their bellies are still small and growing. After feeding them, we tried to get some burps out of them. That was very time-consuming because sometimes it took forever for a burp to come out. When I wasn't feeding with them, I was in utter amazement at how beautiful and perfect they were. I couldn't believe that I had produced two such precious little miracles. I was also still in awe I was a mother! Their personalities showed from the beginning. I had one twin who loved to snuggle and the other twin who was so independent! He would just sleep and stay in his baby cart.

The first night after the C-section, I couldn't move out of the bed by myself. They placed a catheter (a thin tube) to keep my bladder empty throughout the surgery. It was held in place until nighttime when I went to the bathroom for the first time. The nurse had to help me change and use the bathroom. That was such a humbling experience. I was grateful for how the nurse took care of me. When I looked in the mirror, I saw my body for the first time after having my boys. It was emotional and even frightening to see my stomach hanging low and stretched. It looked like a deflated balloon. I didn't want my stomach to stay like that. Thankfully it didn't! The female body is an astonishing creation. The uterus goes through the phase of shrinking back to size after a baby. Breastfeeding also helps with shrinking the uterus. I was super grateful to have my boys with me, but I couldn't help feeling insecure. My body looked like nothing I've seen before. I handled it with grace and tried not to focus on it too much. The nurse was friendly and told me I looked great after having twins. I didn't believe it until some days went by, and my stomach shrunk some more. It's crazy the things you don't know as a new mom that you would experience. There is so much preparation for the new babies, but I think preparation for mommy postpartum is crucial also because the new mom shares so much of herself as soon as her baby arrives. Her entire world is centered on her child. If the mother is nursing, she is sharing her physically body. Emotionally she is concerned about being a good mother. Mentally, her brain is consumed with thoughts about her newborn. The mother also loses sleep. Not to mention her hormones are all over the place. It is a time when the new mother may feel depleted in every way so it is important to be ready for this time as much as possible.

I remember being so sensitive the first few weeks of my babies' lives. I just wanted to do everything right for them. Honestly, I still am sensitive and protective over my sons more than a year later. I think that's a part of being a mother. The three days I stayed at the hospital, I rode the waves of being a new mother and recovering from a C-section. I had to deal with barely having any privacy at the hospital with nurses, doctors, lactation specialists, and insurance employees coming in continually as I breastfed or tried to rest. My sons had to get newborn screen tests and car seat safety checks. I disliked that the boys' father and I couldn't sit in on the screening and reviews, but I prayed for them when they weren't in my sight! I didn't allow my sons to get vaccinated besides the vitamin K shot for circumcision. My spirit and research made me decide not to vaccinate my sons! I wanted to raise my boys holistically and naturally. I read about too many side effects that can come from vaccinations. In my heart, I knew I made the best decisions for my boys. Thankfully I had zero issues or confrontations with the doctors regarding my decision not to vaccinate.

On the last day at the hospital, I discovered the DO NOT DISTURB sign. After finding it, I used it most of the day. I was mentally preparing myself to go home to be a mother of twins for the first time. I felt equipped with the mind, body, and spirit for this new motherhood journey. The following day I made sure the boys and I were packed and ready to go home. It was emotional. I came in pregnant and was going out with two newborns.

It was a little overwhelming getting unpacked when we got home, but their father and I worked well together. We each changed a baby, and as I breastfed or pumped milk, he made sure everything the babies and I needed was in reach. My partner also came home for a couple hours to make sure the house was clean when we returned. I appreciated coming home to a cozy home after being in a hospital for three days. I did have to keep the boys on the same eating schedule they had when we were at the hospital. I have feedings every two to three hours. It seems like I was feeding them all day, every day. I had the challenge of finding the time to do anything else. When I wasn't in nursing, I was pumping. I also had to find time to eat and drink and get some form of rest when I could. The first night after we got settled, my partner's mother came over to help, to allow us take a beneficial nap. We didn't even go to sleep, but we could relax without doing something for the babies. It was like they were the only thing on our minds. After his mother left, we were up every two to three hours like clockwork. If one baby wasn't up crying, the other would wake up crying. We alternated who got the baby, so that's when the pumped milk came in handy because my partner helped me bottle-feed one of the babies when I was trying to rest.

God's Grace over a Diagnosis

On the second day home, we had to take the babies to their first pediatrician appointment. They have quite a few appointments in their beginning life stages to check weight and development. The nurse asked questions about the baby, and the doctor went over newborn screening results. My babies came out healthy and a good weight for twins. I was highly grateful for that and no NICU time. After the nurse did their weight check, the doctor came in to talk to the boy's dad and me. She said everything looked great in the newborn screening, besides one thing. They saw that both babies tested positive for Sickle Cell SS.

Sickle cell is a genetic blood disorder or disease caused by an abnormal form of hemoglobin. When the sickle cells block small blood vessels, the organs are deprived of blood and oxygen. When oxygen isn't following, a pain crisis can occur (Medicine Net, 2018).

When the doctor told us that news, I instantly burst into tears and rocked my sweet baby I had in my arms. Their dad shook his head. No parent wants to hear anything serious about their children, especially after only knowing their babies for five days. I didn't get any test ran when I was pregnant, so I had no clue my sons could inherit the sickle cell trait or blood disorder. Their dad and I didn't know we carried the sickle cell trait in our genetics. No one we know of in our family has sickle cell. As we tried to digest this news, the doctor went on to talk about how serious it was and all the bad things that could happen. Even though this was a hard pill to swallow, I felt the presence of my angels.

I barely knew about SS, but I did remember seeing a girl named Joy from high school talking about it on social media. She spoke about how healthy and good her children were doing because she treated them naturally. As the doctor was talking, I looked at her earrings, and they said JOY.

I took that as an unmistakable sign from the Divine and angels to learn about natural healing to manage SS. After seeing those earrings, I asked the doctor about a natural way to manage SS. She said she had zero knowledge of any natural methods, but I told her I knew someone who did. The doctor then said to find out about it and let her know. She said there wasn't any cure for SS and they would need to take penicillin twice daily for immunity. Supposedly studies say that SS diagnosed individuals have weakened immune systems. I didn't get a positive feeling about penicillin. I turned my head to the right, and there was a sign on the wall that said trust my instincts. The doctors prescribed them penicillin and said she wanted to do one more test to make sure the diagnosis was correct.

The car ride home was filled with mixed emotions, but I told my children's father that I would take care of them naturally if the results don't change. I instantly messaged Joy on Facebook and told her about the situation. I also asked her to tell me how she keeps her children so healthy. She messaged back with so much information on SS and how to take care of it naturally, so my children could thrive. She even told me about a book that explained another mother's journey into natural healing for her son diagnosed with SS. His testimony was that once he started taking herbs, vitamins, probiotics and ate a healthy diet, he didn't have any SS complications for ten years! He only had an issue the first year of his life before taking herbs and only doing what the doctors told her to do. That's when the mom did research and took matters into her own hands. When I heard her and Joy's testimony, I instantly knew my sons would be okay. I had and have extreme faith. I knew if God could do it for them, then He would do it for my children if I followed the signs and guidance.

After speaking to Joy, I went and did my research. I came across this whole Sickle Cell Natural Journey page on Facebook, and it was another answer to my prayers. The page was a whole group of people who managed SS naturally; we share regimens, testimonies, and support. The mother and creator of that page shared her son's unique testimony of having ZERO Sickle Cell issues for two years because of his natural lifestyle. God was giving too many signs. I followed the guidance, and my sons have been doing AMAZING and are incredibly healthy with zero complications.

Fast-forward to a seventeen-month hematology appointment: We were so blessed to find out that our sons have hereditary persistence of fetal hemoglobin, which protects them from Sickle Cell diagnosis. I was so grateful for God's grace. Even though my babies were delivered from Sickle Cell, the diagnosis taught me that nature has a cure for everything, even if Western medicine says there's no cure. That goes to show that it's essential to do research and take matters into your own hands regarding your health and that of your loved ones. I even came across a study from Dr. Sebi that mentioned that "if you take care of your health and live on an alkaline diet, no illness could survive in an alkaline environment." Diseases manifest from mucus, inflammation, stress, and malnutrition in the body. I am convinced that there is a low chance of any mental or physical illness affecting the body if we take care of ourselves holistically.

Chapter 10

Healthy Postpartum

As you have read so far, a lot had transpired during my first week of motherhood. Hearing and learning about my son's diagnosis made me even more health-conscious, not only for them but for myself. Before discovering the wonderful news of protection against the disease due to them having hereditary persistence of fetal hemoglobin, I stayed positive and full of faith.

My postpartum was not like any everyday experience for sure. I was a new mom of twins, and on top of that, I had to learn about how to protect my children from a diagnosis holistically. My motherhood journey only forced me to be stronger mentally, physically, and spiritually.

I noticed myself being randomly moody, and I didn't understand why. I'm so happy that I made a plan on how I was going to handle being a new mother. When things got tough, I went to my self-care routine to make sure I took time to meditate whenever I could, which wasn't much in the newborn stage. Sometimes I would only get five or ten minutes to myself. Still, I used the time that I had wisely. I prayed a lot and used positive affirmations. I also watched my favorite spiritual teachers and listened to uplifting music when the fatigued kicked in. I ate healthier meals to increase my energy. Sometimes eating was a struggle because I felt I was constantly nursing or cleaning up the house. When I wasn't eating enough, I felt weak, so I had to make sure I nurtured and nourished my body with food and water. I also made sure when I felt weak and tired to ask for help from my partner or mother. It is so important to accept help from any close family member who offers. During the newborn phase, all help is beneficial. Even if it's someone just bringing something from the store for you. I would have allowed the boys' grandmas to watch the babies while I took a nap.

After the six-week mark, I started back working out, doing light yoga, or walking. I moved too fast and started to lift light dumbbells and re-strained my neck that I had previously healed in the past. But this taught me a lesson to slow down and love my body unconditionally. Sometimes loving your new mommy body isn't easy—especially with the hormone shifts. I remember getting the baby blues the first week home just because it was an adjustment to a whole new life, and I had a lot to take on at that moment. I was also madly in love with my sons at the same time. It is very typical for moms to have mixed feelings and mood swings. The life that the mom had before is no more, and she's learning about a new life of motherhood that's just beginning. The baby blues feeling didn't last long; it was just the first week for me. I tried not to stay in my feelings too long because I had to focus on learning how to take care of my children the best way. I was just so happy and thankful they were so healthy. In every part of my journey with my sons, I'm delighted and grateful to be able to take care of them. I feel that is a perspective new moms should embrace—being thankful for the energy to take care of their children and also being grateful for healthy children. Being a healthy mother and having healthy children is an extreme blessing. Keeping your thoughts focused on the major blessings will help you overcome the stress from the day-to-day work that comes with motherhood. Also, make sure you do some form of self-care every single day. It doesn't matter if it's only ten to twenty minutes—it's still something for yourself. It can be whatever brings you joy, peace, health, and well-being. My self-care will always be consistent with me eating something healthy, making time to meditate, moving my body, and spending time in nature. It is also beneficial for moms to spend a little bit of time away from their babies—even an hour away going to the grocery store will give the mama a break and some much-needed time for herself. As the babies get older, it will get easier for you to make time to break away or get a babysitter to watch your children.

On some of my self-care days I would get a Reiki healing from a practitioner or do one on myself since I am Reiki Master energy healer. Reiki is an energy healing modality that increases your overall state of health and way of living. In a Reiki session, energy is being sent to each chakra to clear imbalances in the mind, body, soul and auric field. Chakras are the main spinning energy centers in our body. The more energy you have, the better health you have. A lot of energy is used during motherhood—especially during the newborn phase. Reiki was very beneficial to my energy during the postpartum period and now as a mom of toddlers. When you are ready to take time away from your baby, be sure to get at least one day or a blocked-out period for yourself. A day of self-care per week is so needed for a mother's sanity. Being the caregiver is a blessing, but it can be a lot on a person if you don't get a break.

Another way to nurture yourself during postpartum is by tapping into your Divine Feminine Energy. Continue to take care of yourself as a woman. Even though you may not always have the time, do things that make you feel beautiful when you can. I kept my eyebrows threaded and wore light makeup around the house some days. I kept up my hair appointments every six weeks for my routine hair trims. Taking care of your beauty enhances your mood and boosts your self-esteem. I tapped into my creativity through dance and listening to music I love. Dancing and music are healing to the soul. They bring you into a state of flow and stress relief, which is needed during the postpartum phases. When my boys were around six months, I slowly started putting my creativity back into my business. Taking care of yourself and investing in your dreams keeps your identity as a powerful, beautiful woman and will you give you an outlet during postpartum.

Healthy Postpartum Tips:

i. Make time for yourself at least 15 to 30 minutes a day to read or relax alone.

ii. Make time to meditate daily and connect to your spirit.

iii. Move your body daily for at least 15 to 20 minutes a day.

iv. Keep your mind positive.

v. Eat a nutritious diet and drink plenty of water.

vi. Take small breaks with house chores and ask for help when you need it.

vii. Get out of the house one to two days a week for a couple of hours.

viii. Spend time in nature with your baby and by yourself.

ix. Count your blessings daily.

x. When things get overwhelming, honor your feelings. After your self-reflection, affirm that you are strong and you are equipped to handle motherhood.

xi. Get Reiki healings for mind, body, and spirit rejuvenation.

xii. Tap into your Divine Feminine Energy to nurture your beauty, creativity, and power.

xiii. Pray daily!

xiv. Enjoy and love your babies daily!

Chapter 11

Holistic Diet Regime

Having a healthy diet that nourishes you and your baby's mind, body and spirit is key to living a healthy and happy life. It is up to us moms to teach our babies about the healing properties of foods, but we can't teach them if we don't heal our diets first. Before having my sons, I was into wellness and was detoxing my body. I had just gone pescatarian before having my sons. I also started fasting and cleansing my body with smoothies and juices. I subconsciously was preparing my body to carry two lives. I noticed a significant transformation in my body when I started eating cleaner and gave up chicken and dairy.

When I was thirteen, I made the conscious decision to give up beef and pork. After I had my sons, I decided to go plant-based vegan to take our health to the next level. Plant-based vegans eat mainly from natural fruit, vegetables, nuts, seeds, and whole grains. I researched how being plant-based has healed diseases or lowered the risks of diseases occurring in the body. Also, God made everything in nature to heal and nurture our mind, body, and spirit. "Behold, I have given you every herb bearing seed, which is upon the face of all the earth, and every tree, in which is the fruit of a tree yielding seed: to you, it shall be for food" (Genesis 1:29). When I started eating alive food from nature, I noticed so many positive changes in my body. My energy increased, and my digestion improved tremendously. Prior to making this dietary change, I had struggled with constipation due to a lack of fiber, and a lack of prebiotic and probiotic foods! It is healthy to have two to three bowel movements a day.

I never thought I could ever have that many bowel movements daily, but since going plant-based vegan and cleansing my body, I do! When I ate a lot of junk food in high school, I would have a bowel moment every one to two days. It used to stress me out because not pooping creates discomfort. Furthermore, whatever we can't digest just sits in our colon and eventually goes into blood or streams. A clogged and backed-up system ultimately manifests into other health issues. When I studied Ayurveda, I learned that solid digestion is the key to good health. Moms need all the nourishment they can get. We give away our energy daily to our children, partners, housework, jobs, and whatever else our lives call us to do.

Breakfast for a Holistic Mom:

Start the day with warm or room-temperature water. Add a lemon or lime to get rid of extra mucus.

Fruit of choice

Smoothie or green juice.

Organic rolled oats with almond butter, cinnamon, almond milk, chia seeds, or flax seeds are a fulfilling breakfast.

Snack:

Green smoothie (kale, spinach, hemp seeds, almond milk, and banana)

Add superfood of choice: moringa, sea moss, or spirulina

Heaviest Meal:

Lunch: Brown rice, lentil, or choice of beans, sweet potatoes, lightly cooked veggies, or fresh salad

Snack:

Oats, granola, trail mix, nuts, guacamole with healthy chips, hummus, or fruit

Last Meal:

Fresh juice: Beet or green juice or smoothie of mixed berries with superfood acai, Camu Camu, sea moss

Drink water throughout the day and after meals. Add liquid chlorophyll for extra energy. Also, chlorophyll boost the immunity, detoxifies the body, and increases gut health.

Holistic mothers take vitamins and probiotics every day.

Vitamins: Vitamin C, vitamin B complex, vitamin D3, K2 and magnesium

Probiotic of choice for solid health and

digestion

Chapter 12

Mommy Bliss

There are many facets of motherhood, but the best part is the infinite amount of pure love you feel for your children. From the moment I found out I was pregnant, my life changed. I instantly had a love for the growing life inside my womb. I knew with all my heart that I would be able to love and take care of my unborn sons. The day I first laid eyes on them, I couldn't believe they were real. I was a mother to two precious human beings! The love I feel for them goes beyond words and understanding; every time I see them and experience them, I think my heart will explode with love. It's so much love for my sons that I don't even know what to do with it sometimes. I cry tears of joy just looking at them growing and developing. The smell of them, the sound of their voices, the softness of their touch on my skin, and the presence of their loving energy all bring me mommy bliss.

The feeling of love from my sons never gets old. Every single day my love for them expands more and more. There's truly no love like the love a mother has for her children. Even on the days that I'm tired and I feel like I can't go on, one look at my sons gives me all the strength and power I need to take care of them and everything else I have to do. It's genuinely Divine. It makes me realize the love I have for my son is the same love that God has for me and all creation—and it's unconditional and everlasting. Out of all the facets of motherhood, enjoy mommy bliss. It is a blessing to be a mother. No matter how challenging it can be, there's always someone wishing they can be a mother. You are well equipped and divinely chosen for your assignment to be a mom. Step into it with

holistic wisdom and joy.